Eat Well with the Reverse Food Pyramid

3rd Edition

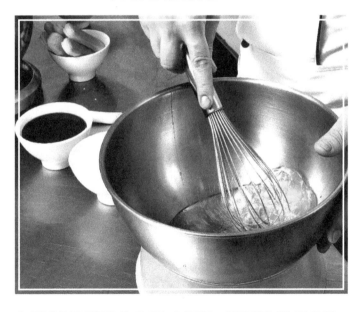

A WORKBOOK AND GUIDE FOR HEALTHY LIVING

By Dr. Diana Pengitore, ND and Dr. Carl Fusco, ND NMD
© The Natural Path, All Rights Reserved

Eat Yourself Well with the Reverse Food Pyramid: A Workbook and Guide for Healthy Living

Copyright © 2018 Dr. Diana Pengitore, ND and Dr. Carl Fusco, ND NMD. All rights reserved. No part of this book may be reproduced or retransmitted in any form or by any means without the written permission of the publisher.

Published by Wheatmark®
2030 Speedway, Suite 106
Tucson, Arizona 85719 USA
www.wheatmark.com

ISBN: 978-1-62787-566-0
LCCN: 2017954711

Contents

Acknowledgments

The Authors

Wish to express their heartfelt appreciation to the following individuals and groups, whose valued input made this book possible:

Dr. Frank Pengitore, Ed.D. for providing the necessary grammatical direction, technical advice, and professional insight.

Mrs. Anna Fusco for her perception, patience, and guidance.

All the friends and clients of The Natural Path who have shaped the focus and scope of this publication through their feedback and loyalty.

"I am feeling so much better in just 6 months! Truly a blessing for me! The plan works."   —*Debbie M. from Texas*

"With the guidance and help of Drs. Fusco and Pengitore, I am able to enhance my diet, find a more organic way of life, which in turn improves my overall health, sleep habits, and stabilizes my emotional well-being... All this in 6 months!"
—*Helen Mary R. from Virginia*

Our Products & Services

Nutritional Guidance

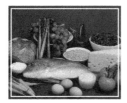

Let us help you make good choices now, and in the future, regarding healthy foods. It is the purpose of this book to get you thinking about what's going in the tank for fuel.

Avoid Inflammatory Foods

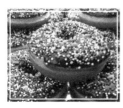

Our main goal with this writing is to steer you away from those foods that propagate inflammation in the body. It is *AVOIDANCE* of these foods that pave the way to well-being.

TSW #1

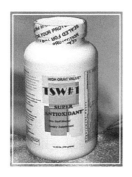

A revolutionary product which supplies a wide range of B-complex vitamins, mega doses of Vitamin C, and high antioxidant content along with enzymes and probiotics, all of which are food-derived. This product is only available through The Natural Path.

Make It Your Own

Name _____

Start Date_____

My Goal(s) is (are);

- ☐ Lose Weight
- ☐ Increase Energy
- ☐ Improve Mood
- ☐ Improve Overall Health
- ☐ Other (list):

  _____

  _____

  _____

  _____

  _____

  _____

  _____

Overview of
"Eat Yourself Well"

Stage 1

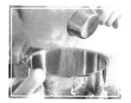

Nutrition 101
Some things about food that you didn't learn in school. A common sense, grass roots approach to keeping the body healthy.

Stage 2

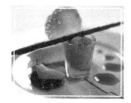

Changing habits, breaking molds, substituting good practices for ones that are not so good.

Stage 3

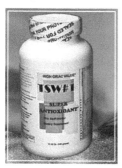

The road to recovery. Don't expect miracles. There will be obstacles in your way. Avoid the pitfalls of fast food and TV ads. Make sure you supplement wisely.

Benefits of this Program

- Weight Loss
- Increased Energy
- Decreased Risk of Obesity, Diabetes, Stroke, and Heart Disease
- Better Management of Stress and Hypertension
- Improved Sleep and Mood
- Prevention of Inflammation and Dehydration
- Better Awareness of Your Own Body's Natural Needs

This book is a self-help guide and program for changing unhealthy eating habits. All can benefit, regardless of health conditions. It is an effective tool when used as directed.

Naturopathic Doctors emphasize the prevention of disease, and we hope that our book will put you back on the road to health. Remember, the change from unhealthy eating habits to healthy ones takes time, practice, and patience. Here's to your health and well-being.

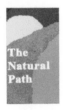

A Workbook and Guide for Healthy Living

Introduction

The road to good health starts with a healthy and well-balanced diet. Because there is such an abundance of food items to choose from, the ***REVERSE FOOD PYRAMID*** displays what ***NOT*** to eat.

By eliminating these poor-quality foods, the body will maintain health and perform better at any age. Realizing that a lot of people do not know much about nutrition, we have identified a void, and taken action in the writing of this book to provide, what we felt, was missing.

Many people take better care of their possessions than they do of themselves. Today's demanding society places loads on our physical well-being. Hypertension, heart disease, diabetes, and obesity are running rampant, and taking people out of a happy, productive life due to avoidable nutritional misdirection.

Early man spent 90% of his time searching, gathering, and preparing his food, so that he could have the energy required to spend the next, and subsequent days, doing the same thing. Today's modern man spends 90% of his day working, worrying, and rushing to do it all again the next, and following days, with little regard as to what is providing his energy.

Processed foods are abundant. Many "foods" are so adulterated with artificial this and artificial that, that they are defined as food by a federal agency (FDA) that has little time to truly analyze their content. We have gone so far from our beginnings as creatures of nature that we have lost sight of how to live in accord with the bounty this planet provides.

For most of us, eating is a secondary consideration. Being creatures of habit, we perpetuate the attitudes and practices taught to us by our parents or those who raised us. The foods we eat, the attitudes we have about food, and the choices we make concerning our meals were taught to us before we could walk or talk.

When attempting to change eating habits, remember that people will continue to revert to the information imprinted during their upbringing. It has been said that it is easier to change a person's religion than to change his or her eating habits.

The diet, those foods consumed on a day-to-day basis, determine the content of cellular make-up, and as such define an individual. The one area in which a person may exercise complete control in life is deciding what to put in the body in order to nourish it. So, that being said, *TAKE CONTROL NOW!* Good luck, and healthy eating.

Eat Yourself Well with the Reverse Food Pyramid

Nutrition 101 (A Primer)

"You are what you eat"! We are all familiar with this saying, but we really haven't given it much thought. Every day, we make decisions about the foods we eat, and over time, these can have a direct impact on our health. Diabetes, heart disease, obesity and hypertension have reached an all-time high in the United States, and it is high time that we start taking care of ourselves. Remember! Your doctor is not in charge of your health—**You are!**

Not all of us have a background education in nutrition, and eating healthy can be a challenge with today's busy lifestyle. Our hectic pace has driven us toward *Fast Food,* for the most part, a processed, high calorie, high fat food choice loaded with sugar and sodium.

Diesel Fuel in your Sports Car

I believe the plan goes something like this: minerals in the soil are absorbed by the root systems of vegetables and fruit trees. The minerals are converted to substances easily assimilated into the human body. Man eats the vegetables and fruits, and absorbs the nutrients. Waste products of man are absorbed into the soil, reabsorbed by the plants, and recycled. Sometimes animals eat the fruits, vegetables, and grasses, then, man eats the animals with the same effect.

If we try to take minerals in the form of supplements that are not food- based, we only poison the body, and add to its toxic load rather than enhance its performance. It's like trying to run a sports car on diesel oil. The fuel is not in the right format, and so instead of high performance, the car runs sluggishly, and over time damage is done to the machine.

Let's take a look at better and healthier foods that can help prevent and/or reverse many health-related conditions.

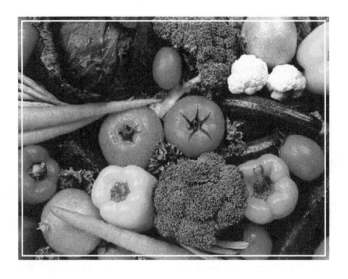

Fresh Fruits and Vegetables

Seventy percent of your diet should consist of this food group, and should be consumed daily. These are considered live foods, as they grow on trees, shrubs and come from the earth and are loaded with helper enzymes, which aid the digestive process. They are loaded with vitamins, minerals, antioxidants, organic sodium, enzymes, and fiber. The body can easily assimilate and digest them, and in return, supply energy. As a matter of fact, a vegetable and fruit day, once or twice a week, would be very beneficial for us. Fresh fruits and vegetables are the forgotten food group.

Cooked, processed (frozen, fried, baked, boxed, canned), and microwaved foods are not as nutritious because a large percentage of vitamins, enzymes, etc. are destroyed during the heating process.

Processed foods may contain added sugar, salt (sodium chloride), artificial flavorings, food colorants, and preservatives. These foods are harder to digest, draining one of much needed energy. Also, these foods can cause inflammation leading to arthritis, diabetes, weight gain, and digestive problems, just to name a few. You may wish to consider vitamin/mineral supplementation at this stage.

The ABCs of VEGs

OK, you've finished your dinner but the vegetables are still on the plate. However, you ate **ALL** the meat.

Here are 26 reasons to eat your "veggies:"

A – Antioxidants	N – Nutrients
B – Beta carotene	O – Omega 3's
C – Chlorophyll	P – Protein
D – D Ribose	Q – Quercetin
E – Enzymes	R – Riboflavin
F – Fiber	S – Sodium
G – Glycerose	T – Trace minerals
H – Hydroxycinnamic acid	U – Ubiquinones
I – Immune support	V – Vitamins
J – Joint health	W – Water
K – Keratins 2	X – Xenobiotics
L – Lignans	Y – Yeast
M – Minerals	Z – Zeaxanthin

NOW... Will you consider eating your veggies?

A Word About Water

Not enough can be said about this vital liquid. It is estimated that the body consists of 80% water; therefore, it requires a daily amount of fresh, clean water (one half your body weight in ounces and no more than 100 ounces per day), in order to function at its best.

Water within the body acts as a vehicle to eliminate waste products, transports nutrients to cells, helps regulate body temperature, and is a major constituent of many of the body's tissues. We have many choices when it comes to water:

- Tap (with added chlorine and fluoride)
- Filtered
- Distilled
- Bottled
- Mineral
- Reverse osmosis
- Well
- Spring
- Rain water

We find that distilled water is still your best choice because it's pure water without added minerals. This allows for nutrients to be carried without competition, and gives waste products a welcome spot for disposal. The pH is an important consideration. Ideally, pH should be around 7.4. Remember, the longer water sits, the lower pH becomes, reflecting an increase in acidity.

Alcohol, coffee, tea, soda, and juice are *NOT* substitutes for water. In fact, these are beverages that can cause dehydration, leading to toxemia and further inflammation within the body. What would happen to the fish in your aquarium if you never changed the water? Eventually, they weaken, and subsequently, die. As we get older, our thirst signal weakens, and gets confused with our hunger signal, resulting in dehydration, weight gain, sluggishness, and little or no energy.

... **"Alcohol, coffee, tea, soda, and juice are *NOT* substitutes for water"** ...

Signs of *Moderate Dehydration* are:

- Darker urine
- Muscle weakness
- Dizziness
- Lightheadedness
- Headache
- Dry or sticky mouth
- Thirst

Signs of *Severe Dehydration* are:

- Increased body temperature
- Mental confusion
- Swollen tongue
- Dark and smelly urine
- Muscle cramps or spasms
- Bounding pulse
- Lack of sweating
- Low blood pressure

If you experience any of these symptoms, call for medical assistance immediately!

Remember, all liquids take the shape of their containers, but in water's case, it may also take on the characteristics of their containers. Soft plastic bottles outgas into their contents, flooding the water with carcinogens and estrogen-like compounds. If you must drink bottled water, try to get it in a glass container.

Most people are dehydrated...

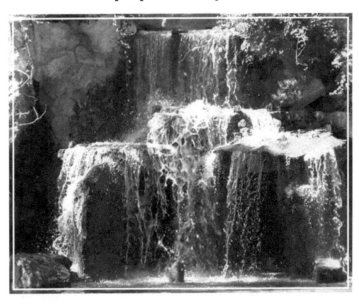

... To maintain good health, drink more water!

Not All Sodium Is Bad

Sodium Chloride and Other Compounds

When doctors put patients on sodium-restricted diets for their blood pressure, what they should emphasize is the limited use of sodium chloride or sodium salts. Salt comes in many forms (table- , Himalayan crystal-, kosher-, and sea salt).

All salt will raise your blood pressure, because salt attracts water to dilute it. Sodium, as an ion, is necessary for regulation of your blood pressure. Many nutrients, including calcium, are not able to cross the cell wall barrier without the aid of a sodium ion. Almost all body functions require sodium. High amounts of salt get eliminated through urination and defecation. Excessive loss, due to diarrhea and vomiting, leads to dehydration.

Organic sodium from vegetables cannot be taken in too high an amount, because functioning kidneys will regulate the sodium level. It is, in fact, the major extracellular electrolyte used to buffer the acidic byproducts of metabolism.

Other chlorides, equally toxic, are the chlorides of potassium, which are often substituted as a safe alternative for table salt. It is not.

Protein

When it comes to protein, meat is not the only source. Protein is found in all foods, some more than others. Animal protein, especially meat, is acid forming and contains unhealthy fats. It can take up to 48 hours to digest, robbing the body of much needed energy. Eating a lighter fare will make you feel better and cause less digestive issues.

Seeds, nuts, fish, eggs, and beans are all excellent sources of protein. Protein provides much in the way of energy. It revs up your cellular metabolism for about 6-8 hours. For comparison, a candy bar provides 15-20 minutes of energy, and a cup of coffee stimulates the body for about 30 minutes.

Amino acids are the building blocks of protein and, contrary to popular belief, we only require 11 grams of protein daily to sustain bodily function. An excess of protein intake leads to an overly acid and over-stimulated system; the kidneys are overloaded and the adrenals are stimulated causing the heart rate to rise and blood pressure to go up. Steroids are released into the system stimulating an insulin response to break down sugar. The liver and pancreas go into high gear and the body's stores of ATP (adenosine triphosphate) are depleted. Your body uses ATP as its primary source of energy.

Body pH is important for the chemistry of life to function at an optimal level. For this to occur, the overall pH of the system needs to hover around 7.4 (an alkaline value). When you take in too much protein, the pH level falls due to the acidity of the protein, and acid byproducts are not adequately buffered. This causes waste products to accumulate along with an increase in oxidative stress. The body attempts to compensate by hyperventilating and producing ammonia in order to re-alkalinize.

... **"Body pH is important for the chemistry of life to function at an optimal level"** ...

Not ALL Fats Are Bad

Remember the "Fat Free" 80's and 90's craze, when we were saturated with media, touting the benefits of a fat free lifestyle? In reality, we were consuming more calories from fat-free and carb heavy foods, and gaining more weight, possibly paving the way for the obesity and diabetes epidemic which is currently all around us.

We should not eliminate all fats from our diet. Fats are necessary for the digestion of our food. They are used as building blocks for hormones, enzymes, and vitamins and provide stability and nutrition for the Central Nervous System (CNS). They pad your organs and supply lubrication for your skin.

Good Fats Are:

- Fats from avocado
- Olive oil
- Canola oil
- Flaxseed oil
- Walnut oil
- Coconut oil
- Oils/fats from fish who live in cold waters (cod, tuna, mackerel, herring, sardines) provide generous amounts of omega 3, 6, and omega 9 fatty acids.

How is oil based paint diluted? With oil, not water. To remove fat from our systems, we need to dissolve it in another fat that washes it out. Drinking more water won't do it. If you use water to clean the brushes (the cells of the body), the paint (bad fats) will only cling more tenaciously.

... "Oils/fats from fish who live in cold waters (cod, tuna, mackerel, herring, sardines) provide generous amounts of omega 3,6, and 9 fatty acids" ...

Milk From Cows

We certainly have been brainwashed about this food. Milk does not do a body good! It thickens mucus, causes bloating, can be hard to digest due to the lack of lactase (the enzyme required to digest it), and is loaded with hormones, antibiotics, and bacteria. In short, it is for baby cows. If you are concerned about calcium and vitamin D from milk, there are other sources to consider such as goat dairy, almond and coconut milk, and dark, leafy greens.

Carbohydrates: Simple /vs/ Complex

Simple carbohydrates (sugar, starches, and alcohol) get utilized immediately, triggering a cascade of enzymatic reactions in the liver. When these are used, the glycogen (another form of carbohydrate) stores in the liver are not utilized, and the body turns them into fat, which is then stored at various places on the body, but mostly around the waistline. Hence, we fight the battle of the bulge!

Complex carbohydrates (whole grains, beans, legumes) are released slowly over time, and allow for the body's glycogen stores to be used, thus preventing fat build up. Eating more of these will help you burn calories at an even pace, and normalize glucose levels in the body.

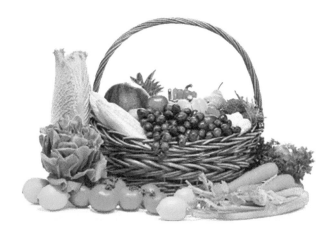

Rich in organic vitamins, fiber, sodium and other minerals

The Nightshade Vegetables

The following are considered nightshades
(after Belladonna, also known as Deadly Nightshade):

- Potatoes
- Tomatoes
- Hot and sweet peppers
- Eggplant
- Cabbage

When eaten raw or juiced raw, certain vegetables can
act like nightshades:

- Broccoli
- Cauliflower
- Kale

It isn't the food that is bad; it's the alkaloids in the plant.
These chemical substances can have an adverse effect
on digestive function, nerve conduction, and muscle
activity, as well as joint health.

Cooking will lower the alkaloid content in the nightshade group by 40-50%. Two alkaloids, in particular, solanine and chaonine have a steroid effect, raising blood sugar, demineralizing joints, blocking cholinesterase (an important enzyme that helps in nerve conduction) raising blood pressure, causing sleep disturbances, and raising anxiety levels.

The good news is not everyone is sensitive to these alkaloids, and for those of us who can safely ingest them, they are a good source of minerals. By the way, Belladonna (Italian for beautiful woman) was given that name for the anti- cholinergic effect on the iris which produced a dilated pupil, thus enhancing a woman's looks back in medieval times.

Enzymes

Foods rich in enzymes (fresh, unprocessed foods) are easier to assimilate, because the body does not require as much energy to extract the nutrients from them. The digestive process for foods lacking in enzymes (cooked, processed, frozen foods) is lengthy and complex, requiring more energy, leaving one tired most of the time.

Remember, the stomach is a muscle, and it requires energy for motion. When enzyme deficient food is consumed, the stomach works overtime to break it down, leaving one energy depleted for the other tasks at hand. A person would consume more of enzyme deficient foods in order to satisfy the body's nutritional requirement, adding to the caloric load and further depleting energy due to inefficient use of the digestive system.

Fiber

According to a study conducted by Tuft's University (2011), Americans do not eat enough fiber. Women require 25 and men 38 grams per day. Fiber is considered "Nature's broom." It is important in the removal of bad fats (LDL), waste products, and mucus from the intestinal tract. Dietary fiber, also known as roughage, is found in whole grains, fresh fruits and vegetables, nuts, and seeds. A healthy balance must be struck, as too much fiber is just as bad as not enough.

Supplementation

There are some nutrients that need supplementation regardless of how good the diet is, for instance, B complex, including folate and antioxidants (especially Vitamin C and reduced L-glutathione). These tend to be used at a higher rate in the body due to their water solubility. Fat soluble vitamins tend to hang around longer before being excreted.

Vitamin C and reduced L-glutathione are master antioxidants. Every day the body needs a new amount of Vitamin C, since it is not synthesized, and it is used in almost every chemical reaction within the body.

It should be buffered and pH balanced at 6.5 to 6.8. Reduced L-glutathione is produced throughout the body, but levels decrease over time with age, illness, stress, and medications. When supplementing glutathione, use only the **reduced** form.

Most vitamins are synthetically produced from petroleum derivatives (oil). These substances are large chain molecules, very often much larger than the cells in which they are to be absorbed. Food derived vitamins or vitamins produced from natural sources are best. Country of origin is important, as well, since some countries are lax in engineering safety protocols during the manufacturing process. It is always best to buy from a local source you trust, and not so much from discount houses on the Internet, as oftentimes the products they sell are closeouts, near expiration, or from unapproved sources. Often, these supplements are stored in warehouses that are not temperature controlled.

What Do Vitamins Do?

Vitamins have many different roles. Some regulate bodily functions (acting as hormones). Some regulate cell and tissue growth. Others act as antioxidants, while the "B" vitamins act as precursors to enzymes and their co-factors work as catalysts in metabolic reactions.

Some work best on an empty stomach due to their water solubility, and some need a fat molecule to transport them across the cell membrane in order to be absorbed. Contrary to popular belief, it may take some effort, but we can get all the vitamins we require from the foods we eat, and not from pills or capsules. Most multivitamin supplements fall far from the mark regarding efficacy. They may contain synthetics derived from petroleum products, or chemical compounds that are larger than the cells that need to absorb them.

Our bodies make some vitamins. The bacteria in the intestinal tract supplies many of the fat-soluble vitamins we require such as A, K, and E. Vitamin D is synthesized from a reaction that occurs when our skin is exposed to sunlight. Contained in that sunlight are UV waves that trigger the synthesis of Vitamin D. Vitamin C must be taken from the diet, as we have ceased to make it for some time due to its high content in fruits and vegetables. Niacin is made from the amino acid tryptophan, and so on.

The B vitamins are depleted in times of stress and exercise. Daily minimum requirements are just what they are, minimum requirements. No studies have been done on what happens when you take more than the minimum, but many scientists believe that supplementing vitamin C is essential during change of seasons and stressful times along with B vitamins.

B-12 injections may be necessary as we age, because your body may stop producing this very necessary vitamin around age 70 when you may develop a condition known as pernicious anemia. Vegans may also suffer with this condition as meat is necessary for its production (fish may also supply the raw materials for synthesis, as well).

Multivitamin compounds are a waste of time and money because they contain fat soluble and water-soluble vitamins, as well as minerals in the form of salts that the body cannot readily absorb. Fat-soluble vitamins (A, D, E, and K) require a fat molecule or micelle in order to be absorbed into the cell; therefore, they must be taken with food.

Water-soluble vitamins need to be taken on an empty stomach because meals interfere with their absorption. Minerals or mineral supplements should always be taken with food. Consequently, half the money is wasted if taken with food, the other half is wasted when taken on an empty stomach. Also, the minerals require so many enzymatic reactions to put them in a format that the body recognizes that the end result is depletion of the very thing that is (supposedly) supplemented. This is especially true for calcium supplements.

All Calcium Supplements Are NOT Created Equal

Salts of calcium, citrate, carbonate, and chloride are not absorbed well. They are, in fact, insoluble mineral salts that provide little to no benefit. Calcium lactate (found in milk) is the most ideal form of calcium, but it is destroyed in the pasteurization process.

Calcium hydroxyapatite is the kind of calcium found in bones, is readily available as a supplement, and is very bioactive. Remember, that calcium carbonate is chalk… the same chalk that teachers use to write on the blackboard.

What Do Minerals Do?

Minerals are mostly metals that help in building tissue, carrying oxygen and other gasses in the body, and buffering chemical reactions to maintain pH. Our bodies operate in a very narrow range of pH, which is the measurement of acid that we can tolerate.

While many of us were bored with chemistry, but loved making that rotten egg smell in class; it is, after all, how we stay alive.

Sodium (a metal) is very necessary to this process, as it provides a means to buffer (maintain a steady pH by absorbing excess Hydrogen ions or Hydroxide ions) created by the physiologic reactions that take place in the body.

Sodium is the main buffering agent used in most of the reactions that take place in the body. When sodium is depleted, calcium becomes next in line. Sodium is used prevalently in the kidneys, and actually helps regulate our blood pressure.

There is a very common trilogy of events due to a lack of sodium that we see in the Naturopathic community, and could be avoided if someone recognized it and increased the dietary sodium intake. The first condition is (1) hypertension caused by inadequate sodium in the diet. This goes on for years until the body starts to remove sodium from the bile salts, causing them to concentrate and become sludge-like, eventually leading to (2) stone formation in the gall bladder. Sooner or later, one of those stones become lodged in the common bile duct, and surgery is performed to remove the gall bladder, the last sodium reservoir in the body. Now that the gall bladder is out, the body must rely on calcium to buffer the acidic reactions of the body, and (3) osteoporosis will eventually follow as that calcium is leeched from the bones and teeth.

Iron is another important mineral in the body (also a metal), which is used to carry oxygen to the cells in the form of hemoglobin. The iron that the body uses MUST be in an organic format like all the rest of the minerals; that is, chelatable. Chelatable minerals are those which can gain or lose 2-3 electrons.

Let's Talk About Minerals

Minerals play a very important role in our lives. Minerals make up our bony skeleton, without which we would have nothing to hang onto. No shape. No form of locomotion. No teeth to chew with, etc. Our muscles would have nothing to move, ergo we could not perform any work, engage in any hobbies, nor accomplish any tasks.

Besides providing structure, minerals move nutrients in and out of the cells. They regulate our blood pressure, and maintain the body's pH by buffering the acidic byproducts of our metabolism. Minerals regulate our heart beat, and are used to make hormones, enzymes, and factor into many of our biochemical reactions.

Most minerals that exist outside of our bodies are in a crystalline form. They exist as large conglomerate molecules (rocks) that cannot be used in our living cells.

Iron, a very necessary mineral to our lives, forms a compound in our blood cells, known as hemoglobin, which is necessary for carrying oxygen to the cells and waste products from the cells in the form of carbon dioxide.

The question is, "How do we get that iron from the soil into our bodies?" And that question also applies to the other minerals, such as zinc, magnesium, copper, sodium, calcium, manganese, phosphorus, chromium, sulfur, chlorine, carbon, etc. The answer is diet.

OK, the obvious answer, but rocks are not part of our diet, nor is it part of any animal's diet that we may eat. So, how do the minerals wind up in our cells? Plants. Yes, vegetables and fruit, and the plants that animals eat. The minerals in the soil are chelated by yeast and bacteria in the root systems of the plants, become a part of the plant, then are harvested by man and prepared and ingested. Our digestive system, through its many enzymatic and digestive processes, assimilates these minerals, perpetuating our lives, and giving us energy.

Some may argue that we drink minerals in our water, but these are not chelated, and only serve to flavor the water and take up space in the liquid. Not very usable. In fact, heavy mineral content in the water makes for stone formation in our hollow viscus organs such as the kidney. Water should be... just water.

Mineral replacement or supplementation cannot be in the form of ionic salts. An example of an ionic salt are those salts which cannot separate at body temperature, such as sodium chloride or table salt, potassium chloride (which is often given to replace potassium that is lost by certain diuretics), and calcium chloride or carbonate which is insoluble and not readily absorbed by the body. The same is true for ferrous metal (magnetic iron). Ferrous sulfate and ferrous chloride are actually poisonous to the body, but iron from food (blood in meat, iron compounds in liver, and cruciferous vegetables) are beneficial and healthy when consumed.

The energy required to separate the metal anion (let's say sodium, potassium, calcium, or iron) from its cation (chlorine) cannot be replicated in our bodies. Enzymatic reactions are just not powerful enough to make it happen.

You see, there are two differing chemistries at work here; inorganic and organic. The primary difference being that organic compounds usually contain carbon, and inorganic compounds do not. Just as you can play cd's in your cd player, they will not play in your tape deck. So it is with your body, minerals must be in a format compatible with your physiology. Vegetables and fruit work great. Meat and fish work well, also.

Magnesium, the Vital Mineral

Magnesium is a very important mineral, and deficiencies seem to be on the rise. Poor diet, a stressful lifestyle, and overuse of prescription and over-the-counter medications (steroids and antibiotics are the worst) all contribute to its rapid depletion. Magnesium can even be depleted by the water we drink if it contains fluoride, chlorine, or heavy amounts of calcium salts (hard water).

Magnesium is known as "The Great Relaxer" in Naturopathic circles, and assists the body in over 300 different chemical reactions. It aids in sleep and relaxation, muscle aches, cramps, spasms, chronic pain, headache, migraine, lower back pain, panic attacks and depression, PTSD, heart health (including rhythm disturbances, vascular tone), and restless leg. Magnesium maintains bone health and steady blood sugar levels, can abate constipation and helps with PMS and pregnancy. It is essential for nerve conduction and central nervous system function. Excessive diarrhea and vomiting will also deplete magnesium. It's a great mineral to supplement after a strenuous workout.

Magnesium is found in the following foods: rye, oats, millet, tofu, beet greens, wheat bran and wheat germ, kelp, seaweed, spinach, nuts, corn, apricots, dates, avocados, figs, shrimp, molasses, brewer's yeast, buckwheat, legumes, monkfish, and brown rice, to name a few.

Supplements of magnesium exist in many forms, mostly as salts. The most common forms are citrates, sulfates, carbonates, and aspartates. Rates of absorption vary.

Craving carbohydrates, salt, and most notably chocolate, is a sign that you may be low in this essential mineral.

A Word About Osteoporosis

Bone mineral density tests are not worthwhile. These tests are money makers for doctors, and do not demonstrate the causes of bone loss. Their accuracy is questionable.

Bisphosphonates (osteoporosis prevention drugs) are made from fish parathyroid hormones. These, and other drugs in that class, are intended to inhibit bone resorption and turnover, yet they cause horrible side effects which include: ulcers, necrosis of the jaw bone, fractures of the femur, blood abnormalities, vomiting, hair loss, etc. In addition to these drugs, patients are often placed on massive doses of Vitamin D (25,000 units a day or higher) which can be toxic.

Bone is a living substance and the minerals require recycling as the cells die; these drugs prevent that. Just as our skin renews itself each month, our bones will do the same. Remember, without organic sodium, calcium cannot enter the cells to make new, healthy bone.

Vitamin and mineral supplements should not be taken in excess! They are, after all, **supplements**... meaning in addition to, not in place of. There is no substitute for a healthy diet.

Organic Foods, Are They Worth It?

People are becoming more health conscious, and the trend toward "organics" is becoming more prominent. A large variety of these items abound, and availability has exploded in the last few years with the advent of markets that specialize in "organic foods."

Mainstream supermarkets have gotten on the bandwagon, as well, and have aisles dedicated to healthy choices and "organic foods." This raises questions for consumers. Are they superior to their non-organic counterparts? Do they offer a health advantage? Are they worth the additional cost?

The USDA defines an organic product as one that contains ingredients that are of 95% organic origin. The "organic" label does not address nutritional content or value. Also, the "organic" classification does not address the way the food was processed. Cupcakes with icing may be listed as organic by USDA definition, but this does not impart to the consumer a healthy diet choice.

It is generally felt that organic foods contain less in the way of pesticides, especially fresh produce; however, if this governs your decision to buy "organic," you might wish to consider guidelines supplied by the Environmental Working Group (EWG), who lists The Dirty Dozen Plus™ (foods with the most pesticide residue) and the Clean 15™ (foods with the least amount of pesticide residue).

A word of caution about buying imported produce. Some countries use pesticides that have been banned in the U.S. When purchasing produce, read the labels for country of origin, and buy appropriately... and wash ALL produce thoroughly before using.

Diets

Let me just put in a word or two concerning diets. There's the Standard American Diet, which can be abbreviated, *S.A.D.* Enough said. And, there are weight loss diets. Diets just don't work. Dieting plans are too restrictive, and are mostly doomed to failure because they eliminate too many foods at once, or drastically reduce caloric intake or portion sizes.

Whenever radical changes are made in eating habits, a stress is created in the body. This stress is digestive and psychological. All new circumstances take about three weeks for the mind to adjust and accommodate. Digestive tracts adjust at about the same rate. This is why, we believe, most diet plans fail in this time frame.

Not only is it necessary for the mind to adjust to these new parameters, but the digestive tract, itself, needs to adjust to the different foods, caloric content, portion sizes, and frequency of meals. Digestive stress can result in bloating, a change in stools, gas, and abdominal pain.

Some diets assume skills that one may or may not possess, such as cooking skills. Preparing food can be quite time consuming, as well, and time is a precious commodity. Other plans offer the food shipped directly to the home, deliciously prepared. Just microwave and eat. Unfortunately, microwaving destroys nutrients (especially enzymes), and the result may be that the box the food came in may contain more nutritional value than its contents!

To sum up, diets are boring, restrictive exercises in frustration that often cause rebound weight gain after the controls come off. We offer a program designed to change your eating preferences, gradually, and over time... something you can *LIVE* with.

Medications and Their Effects on the Body

They may help with pain, but they do not reverse the inflammation. In fact, they may add to the already existing toxic state of the body, and can have many side effects. Medication, over time, will deplete vitamins and minerals from the body; therefore, it is vital to eat a healthy diet, with an abundance of fresh fruits and vegetables, to replenish this loss of nutrients.

Proton pump inhibitors (PPI's) cause the pH in the stomach (the acidity of stomach acid) to increase, that is the environment of the stomach is made more alkaline, inhibiting the breakdown of protein, which is largely digested in the stomach at a very acid pH (1 – 1.5). To further complicate things, long term use of this class of drugs causes the pituitary gland (the body's master gland) to secrete excessive amounts of serum gastrin (a hormone that tells the stomach to produce more acid). High amounts of serum gastrin have been linked to the formation of gastric carcinoma.

Common side effects are headache, abdominal pain, nausea, diarrhea, vomiting, fever, and upper respiratory tract infection. Some severe reactions that may develop over long term use, and are greater in people over 50 years of age are: blood dyscrasias, pancreatitis, fractures, hypomagnesaemia, and Stevens-Johnson's syndrome (a life-threatening condition characterized by bullous lesions resembling pemphigus, hives, and collapse).

A Sweet Topic

Just a word on getting some sugar in your coffee. There are two types of sweeteners available for use, natural or artificial. Artificial sweeteners abound, and are found in a myriad of products that tout "healthy" or "diet" on their labels. They are neither.

Most "diet" drinks and foods contain either aspartame or sucralose. These are truly bad in many ways. Although they are sweet, they provide little health benefit in the long term. These sweeteners cause the body to move into a survival or starvation mode because of their sweetness without calories. The body hoards fat, believing that it is starving, and gains weight over time.

Other problems with these sweeteners are their metabolic by-products. Formaldehyde and methyl (wood) alcohol, at less than body temperature, are products of the breakdown of aspartame. With sucralose, the jury is still out, but combining bleach and sugar can't be healthy, and that's how it's made. Three select hydroxyl groups on the sugar molecule are replaced with chlorine molecules.

Thus far, sucralose has been shown to reduce beneficial microflora in the intestinal tract, increase fecal pH, and increase inflammatory factors in the body, limiting the bioavailability of certain nutrients and drugs metabolized in the liver. These products should *NOT* be allowed on the market.

The American public is becoming more obese as time goes on. "Hungering" for something that can be put in their coffee to wash down the morning cheese biscuits with hash browns that will not give them any extra calories seems as oxymoronic as having a diet soda to wash down a banana split after a four- course meal. Fifteen calories are saved at the expense of three thousand.

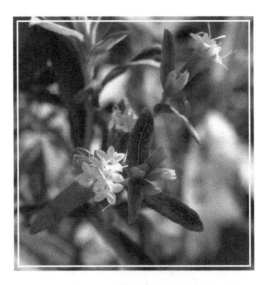

Stevia Gymnativum

Natural sweeteners are just what they are. Yes, they do provide some calories, and are problematic for diabetics. What is the alternative?

Excellent natural sweeteners are Stevia, monk fruit extract, and xylitol. Stevia has negligible effects on blood glucose levels and is perfect for those with diabetes. Similar results are found with monk fruit extract and xylitol.

Stevia belongs to the Asteraceae family of herbs, one of about 240 different species, first discovered for its sweetness by a Swiss botanist (Moises Santiago Bertoni) in 1899. It was later researched by two French chemists (M. Bridel and R. Lavielle) in 1931, who isolated the glycosides that gave the herb its sweet taste, and further refined it into two compounds, stevioside and rabaudioside, 250-300 times sweeter than sugar. Rabaudioside A is available under many different trade names in the United States: ***Only Sweet®, Truvia®, Rebiana®, Pure Via®, Reb A®, and Sweet Leaf®,*** to name a few.

There's always sugar, but refined is always a poor choice over natural, raw cane. At 15 calories per teaspoonful, it can add up to a larger waistline in no time. Most people are taught to eat sweetened foods. Remember that vegetables and fruit are naturally sweet, so why augment these with syrups (water and sugar) and go about dipping strawberries in sugar? The true challenge is the unlearning of bad habits. And that's what this book is designed to change.

Sugar Traps

There are foods out there that we never consider when we think about cutting down on sugar. These are foods that are especially significant to those with diabetes. Sugar is something we are taught to like at an early age and, sometimes, we find it hard to pass up because it is usually associated with a good memory (something we were given as a reward), or a holiday (Christmas, Easter, Halloween). Family get-togethers hold another association with sweets. Who can forget Aunt Martha's apple pie?

Despite the good memories, sugar is, after all, highly inflammatory, calorie intense, and calcium depleting. Without sugar, we cannot produce energy. It's all about balance. However, you never need to eat anything sweet in order to make sugar in your body.

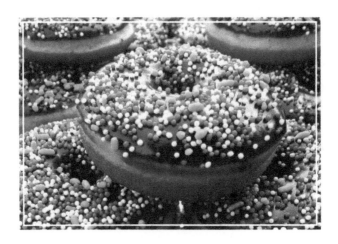

Here are some sugar traps:

- Peanut butter
- Catsup (ketchup)
- Milk (98% carbohydrate)
- Root vegetables (carrots, beets, turnips, parsnips, potatoes)
- Dried fruit (drying process concentrates the sugar content while decreasing fiber)
- Energy bars/protein bars: **READ LABELS!** Some have as high as 24 grams of sugar per serving.

Highest sugar content in fruit:

- Banana
- Mango
- Pineapple

Cut back on these if high glycemic foods are problematic for you. Stay healthy.

A Radical Point of View...

It's always a radical thought, opinion, concept, or idea that tends to throw folks into a tailspin. The same thing happens in the body, but the players are a wee bit different. We're talking about chemical radicals on which the body thrives. Radicals are charged molecules that steal electrons from stable molecules.

This process is called *oxidation*. Oxidation of metal is known as rust. The opposite happens when a molecule with a positive charge is neutralized by gaining an electron. We say it is reduced. Reduced free radicals arrest the oxidation process, and promote longevity and overall good health.

Free radicals are formed every second we are alive as byproducts of our metabolism. Good foods, high in antioxidants or charged with a lot of electrons, are necessary for us to stabilize or neutralize these little "pac men" in our bodies, who chomp away at stable molecules and steal their electrons with a vicious, often domino-effect to the detriment of one's well-being.

Antioxidants are found in a wide variety of foods; i.e.: berries, citrus fruit, cruciferous vegetables, some spices (curcumin and turmeric), carrots and pumpkins (which are great!). Their potency is increased when consumed fresh and uncooked.

What do antioxidants do? Antioxidants are also known as the anti-aging compounds, prolonging cell life and aiding in cell renewal. They also help ease inflammation and detoxify by attacking free radicals. Antioxidants promote healthy brain function and clarify thought processes, enhance heart and eye health, modulate immune response, and provide digestive health benefits.

To reap maximum benefits, it is always best to eat whole foods fresh and raw or lightly steamed. Strive for minimal processing. When antioxidants are taken in this way, they are excellent cancer fighters.

Antioxidants work by supplying electrons and by breaking the chain of free radical, oxidative stress in our bodies. Vitamin C is a great supplier of electrons in a water- soluble format, and Vitamin E is the greatest supplier of electrons in the fat-soluble format. Glutathione is the primary intracellular electron donor.

Antioxidants hold the line against damage to our DNA and the cell, itself. Disease states in the body always trigger an oxidative stress that can show up as faulty cell formation further down the line, resulting in "autoimmune" conditions or aberrant cell division and cancers in an attacked organ.

Remember that we are constantly staving off the attacks of these free radical invaders from our atmosphere (fires, smoke, dust), radiation (the sun, TV, cell phones, microwave, high tension wires), and pollutants in our water and food (food colorants, artificial flavorings, chlorine, bromine, fluorine, bacterial toxins and contaminants, viral DNA and RNA interference). "Aging" (for us) is like a car "rusting" in a junkyard.

Okay, so how do we fight back? Simple. Eat foods and take in nutrition that is high in antioxidant content. Berries, colorful foods, foods high in Vitamins C and E. **ORAC** (Oxygen Radical Absorbance Capacity) values give an indication of a supplement's antioxidant content.

It's pretty straightforward. The higher the ORAC value, the better the food or supplement. Next, consider calorie restriction. Avoid unnecessary calorie loading which leads to an abundance of free radical formation.

Last, cut down on inflammation. Keep teeth in good shape! Low grade infections in the gums and connective tissue surrounding the teeth supply gazillions of free radicals, and therefore increases oxidative stress to the system. See the dentist for a check-up at least twice a year.

Take B-complex and folate supplements daily to stave off oxidative stress in the arteries while nourishing the nervous system. Don't smoke or imbibe alcohol excessively (or at all!). Don't eat processed or microwave cooked foods. Drink adequate amounts of fresh, clean water. This will keep the cells bathed in a broth filled with nutrients while allowing waste products to be carried away. Eat whole, natural foods that are high in antioxidant content (p. 23).

Limit medications (talk this over with your doctor). Use natural sweeteners when needed. Avoid "American" (or manly) foods. It isn't necessary to put bacon or cheese on everything (especially ice cream). Keep calories down, and take in adequate fiber. Move the body. Exercise daily! Follow the guidelines in this book. OK. So, now you know.

Caution, Microwaves Ahead...

Today our lifestyle is fast-paced and hectic. Many times, we reach for the microwave to heat our food, oblivious to the dangers that lurk there. Microwaving food causes it to reach high temperatures very quickly, from the inside out. Because most food contains water, this method of heating is very efficient, as water consists of a polar molecule (a charge on one end and an opposing charge on the other). This results in dielectric heating. Microwaves in use today employ a magnetron tube, generating a frequency of 2.45 GHz (gigahertz), at a wavelength of 12 cm., of non-ionizing radiation. Microwaves are, in fact, a form of electromagnetic radiation.

From a health standpoint, microwaving is associated with cancer and now heart disease. This form of cooking destroys the enzymes in food, and renders them useless strains on our digestive systems.

The latest trend by baby food companies employs the option of microwaving infant formula and baby food. Newborns and toddlers have under developed digestive systems, and microwaving breast milk can create toxins out of normally nourishing amino acids. The same goes for formulas and toddler food.

There are many learned biochemists who feel that enzymes in food are not necessary for their digestion, as the body produces its own enzymes, but we feel that thinking outside the box is necessary from time to time, and what science fails to consider is that enzymatic action from the foods we eat help digestion and energy levels. When "live" (enzyme rich) foods (fresh fruits and vegetables) are consumed, their breakdown starts from bite one. By the time they enter the stomach, digestion is near complete, and by the time they reach the duodenum, little, if any, digestive enzymes produced by the pancreas will be needed. This saves mitochondrial produced ATP (adenosine triphosphate). ATP is the fuel on which our bodies run (energy).

Waking up tired, or being tired all the time, may very well be linked to the amount of digestive energy spent on foods which use more ATP to digest than is produced. If you lack energy, or feel tired all the time, it may be because of this.

Fasting and Juicing

Many people have come to enjoy the benefits of fasting for increased energy and weight loss, when coupled to an exercise regimen. As with everything in life, balance and moderation are key. The American way seems to be, "if a little bit is good, then a lot must be terrific!" Not so, in this case.

First, there are many misconceptions about juicing. Many people have been sold food processors that promise the same or superior results as a juice extractor, but it simply isn't so. These machines are excellent at pulverizing foods into a liquid state, but the foods are not "juiced." Juicing gives you a liquid sans pulp, which enhances nutrient absorption without much digestive effort. Also, many of the enzymes are transferred along with the juice without the interaction on the pulp. In certain instances, this can be extremely anti-inflammatory.

Second, many people drink their juices as they come out of the machine. This is wrong, as the concentrates can be rough on the digestive tract. It is always worthwhile to add, at least, as much water as there is juice yield in order to dilute the juice to avoid overstimulation of the digestive mechanism.

The way juicing works (at least, in theory), is to lighten the load on the body, thus saving energy normally used for digestion, and diverting it to other uses. The average Kreb's cycle produces 36 or so units of ATP (Adenosine Triphosphate), which is the currency of energy that the body uses. EVERYTHING that goes on in our bodies is paid for in units of ATP. Hair growth... so many units, blinking of eyes... so many units, breathing... so many units, Heart beats... so many units, and so on down the line, but digestion?!? For some, it's a 24 -hour process! In fact, the digestive system is almost always active, using up that ATP that we want to use for fishing, shopping, walking, playing the banjo, and bowling. I've been told on many occasions, "Doc, I'm just tired all the time. In fact, I wake up tired!"

This is a prime example of squandering energy units on the digestive process when conservation of energy is actually required. In my 42 years as a medical practitioner, this was the rule, and NOT the exception. A variation of this theme occurs when a high protein content meal is consumed within six hours of bedtime. As protein is primarily digested in the stomach, that muscle stays active over the next 8-10 hours contracting and mixing its contents with the acid that is present. Aside from this, that acid is required to be at full strength in order to cleave the polypeptide macromolecules into their constituent protein chains, and then into their component amino acids.

Taking proton pump inhibitors can be very detrimental to this process. The only indication should be for ulcers or Barret's esophagus. After age 40, stomach acid production begins to decline naturally, so the "reflux" is probably dyspepsia (not enough stomach acid) and the proton pump inhibitor only weakens stomach acid even further, causing an increase in serum gastrin levels (associated with gastric carcinoma) and causing digestive stress on the pancreas for enzymatic breakdown of proteins, perhaps stressing that organ to the point of exhaustion. The pancreas also secretes insulin from the islet cells, and when the pancreas runs out of juice (literally), this may trigger the onset of diabetes. A leaky gut situation ensues when undigested protein enters the circulation and evokes an antibody response. New food allergies are the clue here.

Fasting should only be done under the guidance of a health care practitioner who is familiar with the physiology involved. Your physiology. Fasts should be individually tailored to the person doing the fast. When you fast, it is a chance to eliminate toxins and save energy.

Fasting can put the body into starvation mode, conserving calories and shutting down organs and systems, and HOARDING FAT! Do not fast because you want to lose weight. There are special fasts that help one to lose weight, but do not participate in fasting without a coach that knows what to expect.

The point to remember is that there are organs using energy all the time, even when you are asleep. These organs can, and do, use up the energy you may want to use for other activities, all due to poor dietary choices.

Get Moving!

We have become accustomed to using the car to go everywhere. Drive-through fast food restaurants have become a part of our daily lives. We sit in the office, take the elevator to the car, drive to lunch, eat our lunch in the car while checking emails and returning phone calls, then drive back to work and sit there until the close of business. At home, many hours are spent in front of the computer or television set. To make matters worse, portion sizes in restaurants have more than doubled over the last 10 years. We are consuming more calories on a daily basis than ever before, and NOT burning them off!

The farmer's breakfast with 2-3 (or more) eggs, hash browns, bacon, sausage, juice, toast, coffee, milk, and pancakes has no place in our techno-society. It's OK for those who spend the day burning calories by putting in a hard, physical day; but, it is not OK for office workers or others with a sedentary lifestyle.

Here are some tips to incorporate a little exercise into our busy lives:

- Walk more
- Walk up and down the stairs whenever possible
- Walk the dog; if you don't have a dog, borrow one to walk

- Park the car a little further away and walk to the restaurant
- Walk a block, a few times a week
- Park further away from shops, work, etc., and walk the remaining distance
- Did we mention walking more?

Aging does not have to be debilitating and painful anymore. By taking charge of our health today, gradually incorporating changes by means of a better and healthier diet, the aging process can be decelerated.

Regular exercise has benefits of its own, and deserves to be extolled all by itself. But whatever you decide, do it on a regular basis... daily would be good... or even more than once a day!

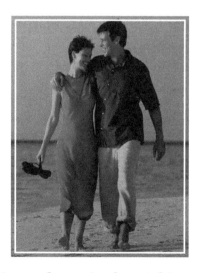

Exercise can be as simple as taking a walk.

Candida

Candida is, simply stated, yeast. There are 52 known species of this yeast which is known to ferment glucose and maltose into gas. The common varieties which are known pathogens (cause disease) are: C. Albicans (most common), C. Dubiensis, C. Glabrata, C. Guilliemondii, C. Kefyr, C. Kruseii, C. Lusitraniae, C. Milleri, C. Oleophilla, C. Parapsilosis, C. Theae (2), C. Tropicalis, C. Viswanathii, and C. Utilis.

Yeast are single-celled organisms in the fungus family, and do not require sunlight as they receive their nutrition from organic compounds such as glucose or fructose. In small amounts, they are, of themselves, nutritious, and are found in breads, pickled items, and other fermented foods. They occur normally in nature and are known to help break down nutrients in the soil for plants to absorb through their root systems. In humans, they are universally present on the skin, and are found throughout the alimentary tract.

We all have candida in and on us. When kept in balance, like all things in our bodies, candida does not pose a problem for us; however, once it overgrows, it takes diligence and a concentrated effort to eradicate. Once balance is restored, it is easy to maintain.

How do they make us sick?

When candida organisms overgrow, they produce
hyphae, a branch, as on a tree. This "branch" penetrates
the mucus membrane and produces irritation. When
this happens on the surface of the skin, you scratch.
Scratching drives the organism deeper into the skin
and into the surface blood vessels located there
(the capillaries) where an antibody reaction takes
place, initiating the body's response to trauma. A
cascade of immune factors is released from the cells
which produce redness, swelling, and pain (burning
and itching). Candida Albicans is the most common
cause of these symptoms. This condition is known as
candidiasis.

But the biggest reason people fall prey to candida
infection is ignorance. Symptomology is vague,
orthodox medicine doesn't believe in candida as the
cause, and they have a pill for that. Problematically,
this type of thinking has led the unsuspecting public
straight into the slaughterhouse. The candida organism
is a great mimic. It has managed to imitate a variety of
conditions which further frustrates proper treatment.
Some of the conditions it may impersonate are asthma/
allergies, eczema/psoriasis, diabetes, ear infections,
sinusitis, digestive issues, multiple sclerosis, and ADD/
ADHD/Autism to name a few.

Some of the earlier approaches to candida have included diet (to starve the yeast), various alternative remedies (oregano oil, EFA's, Acidophilus and other probiotics, caprylic acid, garlic, various vitamins and minerals, and anti-oxidants.)

Medical approaches (when recognized as thrush or vaginitis) consist of various antifungals given topically or as troches, or even given internally as very expensive pills (e.g.: Diflucan $22.45 per tablet, in generic form).

The drawbacks to these methods were that they didn't go far enough, or were applied ineffectively. Candida does develop resistance to anti-fungal preparations over time, no matter how much they cost, and many, if not all, of the systemic medications are toxic to the liver; added to this are the widespread use of antibiotics and steroids which suppress immune response and alter gut flora, further enhancing the environment in favor of candida over growth.

In 1953, Dr. Orian Truss, MD recognized a condition he termed "antibiotic syndrome", and later wrote a book called, *The Missed Diagnosis.* In 1986, Dr. William Crook wrote a book called, *The Yeast Connection,* which offered his solution, the candida diet.

How do you know you have it?

There is a saliva test that is touted as the "sine qua non" for home/self- diagnosis. This entails expectorating into a vessel filled with cold water and watching for trailers of spittle (like the tentacles of a jelly fish) extending down into the water. This is inaccurate and will be "positive" in about 70-80% of those who take the test. Remember, candida is normal to the body in everyone and is prevalent throughout the integument (skin) and alimentary tract. And, the mouth is part of the alimentary tract.

As there are no definitive tests to demonstrate a candida infestation, this condition is diagnosed chiefly through a provider's clinical intuition. There are many clues that will lead a clinician to consider the diagnosis of candidiasis. Do not be misled by the myriad of tests and procedures that abound. Most have no scientific basis, and the ones that are science- based are inconclusive, at best. Treatment of suspected candidiasis is simple and effective, and does not involve invasive procedures.

How is it reversed?

One must keep in mind that this condition, as with most natural methods, takes time to reverse. However, candida infestations respond quite well to the restoration of the body's ecological balance by reducing the intake of starch and sugars.

Anyone with suspected candida symptoms should be individually assessed and begin treatment immediately. A candida diet is necessary for the first 2-4 weeks to keep growth of candida organisms in check. pH must be restored,
and an anti-candida protocol instituted. A well-balanced probiotic must be part of the plan.

The rule of thumb is one month of treatment for every year of the problem. Candida is such a subtle condition that many will not know the duration of their illness; therefore, we aim for reversal of symptoms plus three months in the management phase.

In many instances, common medical complaints and a visit to your doctor can create the ideal environment for a yeast problem. Let's take a common scenario. You have a cough, and it has been hanging around for two weeks. You decide it's time to see someone about it. You call your doctor's office and make an appointment. You check in, and are eventually seen and evaluated by a health care provider (MD, PA-C, or NP). You are diagnosed with bronchitis, and given a prescription for antibiotics. Most health care providers are aware of the role antibiotics play in killing off good bacteria with the bad, but for some unknown reason they never mention that the good bacteria must be replaced with the help of a probiotic.

Often, bronchial type coughs are treated with a steroid spray to calm the irritation in the bronchial mucosa. Steroids do many bad things with regard to yeast, such as: Acidify the body, raise cortisol levels, thereby increasing blood sugar levels (which yeast love), and suppress the immune response.

Now, the deck is really stacked in favor of the yeast, and the practitioner you consulted never mentions anything about the diet, which can further feed the yeast, perpetuating and/or exacerbating the problem. The lesson to take away here is to make the provider aware of the side effects of the medication, and to advise the provider that a good probiotic will be a lot better than, "just eat some yogurt."

Stay healthy.... And informed.

Symptoms

- Fatigue and foggy thinking
- Sugar cravings
- Abdominal bloating/pain
- Cannot lose weight no matter what is tried*
- Vaginal irritation/discharge
- UTI's
- Rashes/itching (especially rectal area)
- Coated tongue/thrush

- Bad breath/foul taste in mouth
- Allergies to foods
- Joint pain/arthritis
- Sinus drainage
- Fungal infections of nails
- Itchy, red eyes
- Hair loss
- Vision changes
- Depression
- Feeling 20-30 years older than you are
- Doctors tell you there is nothing wrong

*Key symptom of candidiasis

If you are experiencing any of the above, remember that candida is a great imitator, and many serious medical problems can be mistaken for candida. Consult your health care providers, and let them rule out more serious conditions before commencing a candida treatment. If, though, the standard treatments for what you have are ineffective or make things worse, consider candida as the cause.

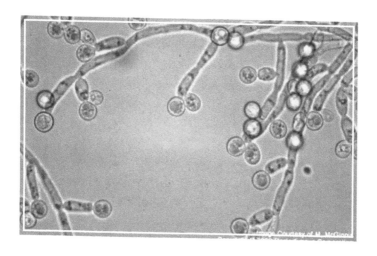

Image Courtesy of M. McGinni

Diabetic Considerations

Diabetes? Now what?!?

You are told you have diabetes. The initial reaction is shock. Is this it? Can it be cured? Am I going to be on medication for the rest of my life? And then- What the heck is diabetes, and why did I get it?

Unlike other conditions where medication is the only means of management, diabetes requires a total involvement and commitment in terms of lifestyle management and change. Chances are this was not anticipated, or it may tend to run in the family. Conventional medicine may blame genetics, but eating habits, learned before the age when you talked and walked, are probably to blame.

What is diabetes? Diabetes, briefly stated, is the body's inability to metabolize glucose correctly, resulting in high blood sugar levels. Uncontrolled diabetes can lead to blindness, heart disease, neuropathy, amputations, chronic infection, and vascular disease, among other serious maladies.

To help with lifestyle management and change, a list of diabetic considerations is included as a quick reference guide:

- Drink more water—at least six, 8-ounce glasses per day. The body cannot function properly without an adequate amount of water.

- Drink traditional green tea; it is high in antioxidants.

- Try juicing with a conventional juicer; no ninja or bullet. Dilute juices with an equal amount of water. Avoid root vegetables. They are higher in sugar content.

- Use stevia, xylitol, or monk fruit extract to sweeten drinks and food. These are 0 calorie, natural alternatives to sugar.

- **DO NOT USE** honey, agave nectar, etc.

- **DO NOT EAT OR DRINK** food or drinks sweetened with Splenda® (also known as sucralose), NutraSweet® (also known as aspartame), or high fructose corn syrup.

- Use a crockpot more often; also, poach, steam, or pan sear your food.

- Eat more whole grains, e.g.: barley, steel cut or old-fashioned oats, or brown rice.

- Eat rye or pumpernickel bread. DO NOT EAT any white flour bread.

- **DO NOT EAT** any white flour baked goods (crackers, etc.).

- Eat more salads and vegetables; use corn, potatoes, and rice in moderation.

- **DO NOT EAT** any dried fruits, bananas, mangoes, and pineapples as they are high in sugar.

- Consider ¼ cup of fruit as an in-between meal snack; eat melon by itself, as it digests rapidly.
- **DO NOT EAT** foods loaded with BBQ sauce and other condiments (use these sparingly).
- **DO NOT EAT** commercial peanut butter, as it is high in sugar.
- Eat more beans, lentils, peas; they are also perfect for crockpot cooking.
- Add chia seeds to your diet (if able), they are high in nutrients and fiber.
- **DO NOT EAT** sugary cereals, e.g. Honey Nut Cheerios®, etc. A good cereal is Kashi 7 Whole Grain Puffs® (unsweetened).
- Use almond milk instead of dairy; aim for the unsweetened variety.
- Add cinnamon and curcumin (turmeric) to your diet. Cinnamon helps regulate blood sugar levels, and turmeric is a natural antioxidant with anti-inflammatory properties that protects the nervous and cardiovascular systems.
- Add essential fatty acids (EFA's) containing Alpha Linolenic Acid (ALA), Docosahexaenoic Acid (DHA), and Eicosapentaenoic Acid (EPA) to your daily diet. The body needs them and cannot manufacture them. EFA's are available from fish-, flax-, grapeseed-, cranberry-seed oil, etc.

- Eat more fish, e.g. salmon, mackerel, cod, sardines, tuna, which provide high amounts of omega 3 and 6 fatty acids.

- Add antioxidants to your diet to protect it from free radical damage, B vitamins to protect the Central Nervous System, and Benfothiamine (a form of vitamin B-1) to prevent nerve and blood vessel damage.

- Read food labels for sugar information. Be aware that sugar grams are listed "per serving" not "by container." Some other names for sugar are: glucose, acarbose, fructose, galactose, and sucrose.

- Add the juice of a fresh lemon to drinking water to help alkalinize it.

Your Healthy Life Begins Here...

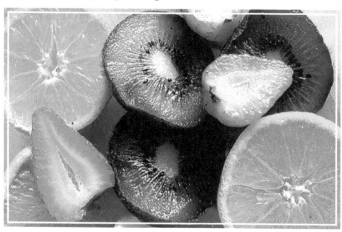

Getting Started

There are components to good health. This program addresses one aspect... nutrition. To use this program efficiently, it is necessary to write down the foods you eat. Next, compare them with the categories listed on The Reverse Food Pyramid, and circle or highlight the ones which correspond. It is here that you must exercise conscious control. Pick a category that is highlighted, and try to eliminate it from future journal entries.

Unlike the old, familiar Food Pyramid, which suggested foods TO eat, The Reverse Food Pyramid is meant as a guide of foods NOT to eat. All foods listed in The Reverse Food Pyramid should eventually be eliminated from the diet, starting anywhere you like. Each week, try to eliminate another category. Keep in mind that we are all human, and will tend to slip. Just do the best you can! Your ultimate goal is to have a clean diary page with NONE of the food categories that are listed on The Reverse Food Pyramid present.

We all know that "DIET" is a four-letter-word. Good health is not a right... it's not a guarantee. But, one thing is sure... it is attainable. The diet needs to be changed in baby steps because radical changes will result in reverting back to old habits quickly.

Throughout this book healthy tips and suggestions have been placed to aid in the quest for a healthy lifestyle. You will find over time that healthier items will end up in the shopping cart and on your table.

Forget all that you have heard about dieting. We are not proposing any diets here.

... "Unlike the old, familiar Food Pyramid, which suggested foods TO eat, The Reverse Food Pyramid is meant as a guide of foods NOT to eat." ...

Rather, think of this as "The UN-Diet." We, at The Natural Path, are committed to your success, and the healthy tips in this book are meant to enhance your journey on the road to a healthy, happier life.

Tips for Healthy Eating

1. Drink more water: ½ your body weight in ounces (as a general rule)

2. Eat lighter fare when eating out (grilled, braised, boiled, steamed)

3. Dilute fruit juices

4. Snack on fresh fruits and vegetables instead of chips, pretzels, candy, etc.

5. If you must snack, eat plain popcorn instead of buttered and salted

6. Eat your food slowly, and chew your food well before swallowing it

7. Wait at least 10 minutes before taking seconds (allow yourself to feel full)

8. Add chia seeds to your diet—an excellent source of fiber

9. Do not eat heavy meals late at night; i.e.: after 8:00P.M., you increase the body's workload on the digestive system

10. Do not eat fruits and proteins together

11. Even fruits and vegetables should be eaten 10-20 minutes apart due to the different enzyme activity required to digest them

12. Purchase a water filtering system

13. Purchase a juicer, and USE IT. Juicing provides nourishment without the body having to work hard at extracting the nutrients

14. See your Naturopath at least twice a year

15. Eat more fiber. You need to move things along

16. Don't starve yourself all day, thinking that skipping meals will save you calories. Your body will go into starvation mode, hoarding calories, and you will eat everything that's not nailed down when you finally DO eat

17. Plan your meals ahead of time, and shop for those meals

18. Never go shopping when you're hungry

19. Eat a good breakfast

20. Decrease restaurant use; you have no control of how the food is prepared

21. Buffets are DEADLY! Avoid them like the plague

22. Decrease TV time. Watching TV promotes the urge to snack. It's your way of interacting with the screen. Conversely, computer time decreases your urge to snack, as your hands are busy (most of the time)

23. Never eat on the run

24. Do not use food as a coping mechanism for dealing with stress

The Reverse Food Pyramid

This is meant as a guideline of what *NOT* to eat!

Try to eliminate categories from these groups every day.

In a few weeks, you will notice an improvement in your **overall health and well-being.**

*Animal Proteins (especially red meat)
Seafood is OK, as a general rule
Dairy Products Except Yogurt and Hard Cheeses (Goat Dairy OK)
*Processed Meats: Cold Cuts, Jerkey, Sausage, Hot Dogs, Hamburgers and Bacon
The Nightshade Vegetables: Cabbage, Potatoes, Tomatoes, Squash (if Hypertensive)

*Bad Fats: Trans Fats and Saturated Fats, Deep Fried ANYTHING
Refined Foods: Flour, Sugar, Salt, Rice, Pastries and Doughnuts
Quick Release Carbs: Candy, Breads, Pastas
Energy Bars/Drinks with High Grams of Sugar

Processed Foods and Fast Foods / Restaurant Fare and Buffets
*Microwaved Foods
Snack Foods
Fried and High Heat Cooked Foods
*Foods That Do Not Look Like They Grew on a Tree Or Came from the Earth

*Foods High in Inorganic Sodium and Sugars/Artificial Sweeteners
Stevia is Acceptable
Artificial Flavorings and Colorants
Condiments

High Fructose Juices *Sodas
Caffeinated Beverages
*Alcohol

*Worst Categories
All these are bad for you, but these are the priority eliminations.

Conceptualized by
Diana Pengitore, ND
and
Carl Fusco, ND NMD

Courtesy of The Natural Path

©2010   No reproduction of this chart, in whole or in part, is authorized without the express, written permission of the author(s).

My Progress at 3 months

Food Categories Eliminated:

_____   _____

_____   _____

_____   _____

_____   _____

_____   _____

My Progress at 6 months

Food Categories Eliminated:

_____   _____

_____   _____

_____   _____

_____   _____

_____   _____

My Progress at 9 months

Food Categories Eliminated:

_____   _____

_____   _____

_____   _____

_____   _____

_____   _____

My Progress at 12 months

Food Categories Eliminated:

_____   _____

_____   _____

_____   _____

_____   _____

_____   _____

Do not use food as a reward for your children or yourself.

Beware of the Holidays! It's OK to slip for the day, but not for the whole month...

Don't feel justified in exchanging good eating habits for bad ones just because "'tis the season".

Suggested Reading and Web Resources

Fit for Life, Harvey and Marilyn Diamond, ISBN # 0-446-30015-2, $7.99 USD; This book is not a diet book, but has wonderful tips on how to eat and food combining.

American Institute for Cancer Research (AICR); New American Plate on www.aicr.org

For chia seeds, a great source of fiber, try: mychiaseeds.com

For everyone, not just diabetics: www.mendosa.com/gilists.htm This website lists glycemic index and glycemic load values

How to Contact Us

We welcome your feedback and success stories, and if you find yourself in the area, please do not hesitate to stop in.

Phone: (757) 478-4455
email: dr_carlfusco@yahoo.com
www.naturalpath-vb.com

References

Aloia, J. F. (1995). *A colour atlas of osteoporosis.* Aylesbury, England: Mosby-Year Book Europe Limited.

Batmanghelidj, F. (2008). *Your body's many cries for water* (3rd ed.). Los Angeles, CA: Global Health, Solutions, Inc.

Diamond, H. & Diamond, M. (1985). *Fit for life.* New York, NY: Warner Books.

Ferri, F. F. (2006). *Ferri's clinical advisor: Instant diagnosis and treatment.* Philadelphia, PA: Elsevier Mosby.

Fiber from grains linked to living longer. (2011, May). *Tuft's University Health & Nutrition Letter, 29*(3), 1-2.

Fors, G. (2007). *Why we hurt: A complete physical and spiritual guide to healing your chronic pain.* Woodbury, MN: Llewellyn Publications.

Harrar, S. (Ed.). (2004). *The sugar solution.* Emmaus, PA: Rodale, Inc.

Hendel, B. & Ferreira, P. (2003). *Water & salt: The essence of life.* Gaithersburg, MD: Natural Resources, Inc.

Joyal, S. (2008). *Diabetes: An innovative program to prevent, treat, and beat this controllable disease.* New York, NY: Wellness Central.

Levy, T. (2002). *Curing the incurable*. Henderson, NV: LivOn Books.

Levy, T. (2006). *Stop America's #1 killer!* Henderson, NV: LivOn Books.

Levy, T. (2008). *GSH: Master defender against disease, toxins, and aging*. Henderson, NV: LivOn Books.

McIlwain, H. & Bruce, D. (2004). *Reversing osteopenia: The definitive guide to recognizing and treating early bone loss in women of all ages*. New York, NY: Henry Holt and Company, LLC

Mitchell, F. L. (2002). *Instant medical surveillance*. Beverly Farms, MA: OEM Press.

Prevention Health Books (Eds.). (1996). *Healing with vitamins*. Emmaus, PA: Rodale, Inc.

Scott, T. (2011). *The anti-anxiety food solution*. Oakland, CA: New Harbinger Publications, Inc.

Somersall, A. (1999). *Breakthrough in cell defense*. Smyrna, GA: GOLDENeight Publishers.

Webb, D. (2011). *Healthy eating: Essential dietary strategies for living a longer & healthier life*. Norwalk, CT: Belvoir Media Group, LLC.

About the Authors

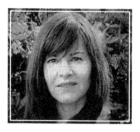 Dr. Diana Pengitore, ND is a Naturopathic doctor who received her graduate training, with honors, from the Clayton College of Natural Health in Birmingham, Alabama. She has a strong background in Homeopathy, Nutritional Counseling, and is a Certified Master Reflexologist.

Born and educated in Germany, Dr. Pengitore is proficient four languages, German, English, French and Spanish. She is currently affiliated with The Natural Path in Virginia Beach, Virginia.

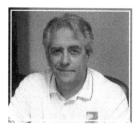 Dr. Carl Fusco, ND, NMD, is a Board Certified Naturopathic Physician. He received his Doctorate in Naturopathy from Trinity College of Natural Health in Wausau, Indiana and his Doctorate as a Naturopathic Medical Doctor from the University of Science, Art, and Technology in Montserrat, BWI.

He is the founder of The Natural Path in Virginia Beach, Virginia, specializing in wellness assessment, Iridology, and Diet and Lifestyle Counseling.

Notes

This page is included for those who love to annotate their books. On the following page, there is an example of a food log. Food logs are instrumental to help you get where you want to be. You may copy this one, and enlarge it in order to mark your progress week-to-week. You may use the reverse side to track blood pressure, blood sugar (if applicable), and any notes on foods and reactions to them.

There is a section at the bottom to track energy, mood, and sleep on a scale of one to ten, ten being the best. If the sheets are placed atop one another, you may easily track your progress from week to week by lifting the previous page just above the weight/energy/mood/ sleep index below it.

Week   Month   Year

	Monday Breakfast	Tuesday	Wednesday	Thursday	Friday	Saturday	Sunday
Lunch							
Dinner							

Snack/Beverages

End of Week Health Check:

	1	2	3	4	5	6	7	8	9	10
Energy										
Mood										
Sleep										

Weight _____